Fat Bombs

A Year of Sweet & Savory Paleo, Fat Fasts, and Gluten Free Fat Bombs: 52 Seasonal Recipes Included!

Table of Contents

Introduction

Congratulations on downloading your personal copy of *Fat Bombs*. Thank you for doing so.

Hearing the words fat bomb could scare the pants off anybody trying to lose weight. But there's no need to worry; these are full of cream cheese, butter, coconut oil, coconut butter, cream, and coconut cream which are actually good for you. Your body takes a longer time to break down fats, so this slows done the breakdown of carbs into sugars. These fats also help to feel you up. If you choose to have a fat bomb for breakfast, then it can reduce your need to snack later in the day.

If you are on a low carb or paleo diet, then the fat will help you power through the day, and it also gives your body something to digest. This will also stabilize your blood sugar preventing any of those nasty side effects.

Now it's up to you to start using these fat bombs. It's not too hard to get started with because recipes are found just about anywhere, and there are 52 in this book. If you don't like the sound of fat bombs, call them energy balls. But instead of them having a bunch of oats and fruits, they have fats and other flavorings. Most of these bombs contain 85% fat. They also tend to follow the rules for gluten free, paleo, ketogenic, and low carb diets.

They may be tasty, but because of their fat content, it makes it extremely difficult to over eat them. They can be savory or sweet, with the sweet ones being the favorite. They will also need to stay refrigerated because of the amount of fat that is in them.

Fixing your fat bombs is extremely easy to do, so let's get to the tasty treats.

There are plenty of books on this subject on the market, thanks again for choosing this one! Every effort was made to ensure it is full of as much useful information as possible. Please enjoy!

Spring

Orange Creamsicle

These treats will remind you of those push-ups that everyone enjoyed as a child. The fat bombs will store well in the fridge but will be more of the consistency of Jell-O. If you want them to be firmer and hold their shape, then storing them in the freezer is probably the best option. Either way, they are delicious.

Yields: 24

Keto, Gluten-Free, Fat Fast

Ingredients:

½ c boiling water

1 pck orange Jell-O, sugar-free

2 tbsps. coconut oil

8 oz cream cheese

3 tbsps. erythritol, powdered

1 c whipping cream

Instructions:

1. Place the erythritol and the whipping cream into a stand mixer and whip them until fluffy.
2. Slice the cream cheese into four pieces and then microwave until really soft, but not to the point that it's melting.
3. Switch the wish attachment to a paddle and begin slowly adding the softened cream cheese.

4. While that is mixing together, place the butter in a bowl and melt in the microwave. Then slowly start adding this into your mixture.
5. Pour the water over the Jell-O and stir until dissolved, about five minutes. Then slowly place this into the mixture.
6. Grab some silicone molds, and pour this mixture into the molds. Place this in the freezer for around three hours before you take them out of the molds.
7. Pop the fat bombs out of the molds, and keep stored in the refrigerator or keep frozen for a nice cold treat.

Key Lime

Florida and spring are nearly synonymous, especially for people who take spring breaks. Two amazing things that come from Florida are key limes and key lime pie, so why not bring this tasty treat to the world of fat bombs. These are perfect little bite sized key lime pies without all the carbs. They are delicious and creamy and a lot of other adjectives.

Yields: 20 – depending on size

Keto, Gluten-Free, Fat Fast

Ingredients:

1/8 to ¼ tsp Stevia, powdered – depends on how sweet you want them

¾ c key lime juice

½ c coconut butter

1 c coconut oil, melted

2 c raw cashews, soaked for at least two hours

Instructions:

1. Place all of the above ingredients into your food processor and mix it up until it has all come together.
2. Pour this mixture into a bowl and let it freeze for 20 to 30 minutes, so it cools off and makes it easier to handle.
3. Take the mixture out and then form it into balls, whatever size you would like, but typically it should make 20.

4. Set these balls back into the freezer for another 20 minutes so that they can harden up. Setting them on a cookie sheet or plate that has parchment paper on it works best so that they don't stick to each other.

5. After they are hard, remove from the freezer. Place them into a storage container and then keep them in the freezer or refrigerator. If you keep them frozen, you will want to let them set out for a bit before biting into one.

English Toffee

Fat bombs really should have a more appetizing name like, little drops of heaven, but since they don't, enjoy them in front of your friends and watch as they stare in amazement that you can eat them and still lose weight. These fun toffee flavors are great breakfast snack or midday pick me up.

Yields: 23

Keto, Fat Fast, Gluten-Free

Ingredients:

3 tbsps. English Toffee syrup, sugar-free

½ c natural peanut butter

¾ tbsp. cocoa powder

4 oz cream cheese

2 tbsps. butter

1 c coconut oil

Instructions:

1. Place all of the above into a pot and stir it together until it becomes smooth and well incorporated.
2. Grab a mold that you like, such as a mini muffin tin, or silicon molds. Pour the chocolate mixture into the mold of your choice and then slide them into the freezer.
3. Let them freeze for a few hours, or until they are completely set. Pop them out of the molds and do your best not to eat them right away.

Place in a container and keep them in the freezer or fridge.

Easter Egg

These cute little Easter eggs will give you a healthy snack, and give your kids something to help you make. They give you the opportunity to have again and decorate them however you want. If you don't want to do the colored coating, you can omit it completely, or dip it in sugar-free chocolate.

Yields: 14

Keto, Fat Fast, Gluten-Free

Ingredients:

1/3 c dark chocolate chips, sugar-free

¼ tsp gray sea salt

5 to 10 drops Stevia

1 tsp vanilla extract

½ c coconut oil, melted

2 c almond flour

Coating:

Easter colors

½ c coconut butter, melted

Instructions:

1. Take a cookie sheet and place a silicon baking mat over it.
2. Place the salt, stevia, vanilla, coconut oil, and almond flour in your food processor and mix it up until it is smooth.

3. Mix in the chocolate chips. Take a tablespoon and a half of the batter into your hands and roll it into a ball. Set it on your cookie sheet and flatten and shape it into an egg. Do this for the rest of you dough.
4. Place the cookie sheet in the freezer for an hour.
5. Place a cooling rack on top of another cookie sheet and place to the side.
6. For the coating, melt the coconut butter and split it between a few bowls, depending on the colors you want to use. Color each with an Easter, inspired color.
7. Take out the eggs and coat one side of the eggs with coconut butter and set on the cooling rack. Once they're coated, place the rest of the coconut butter into Ziploc bags, one bag for each color, and snip off the corner. Drizzle the colors over the eggs. Get creative with this.
8. Place the eggs into the fridge for an hour.
9. They should stay cool in a container in the fridge for about five days. If you freeze them, they keep for a month.

Matcha Coconut

If you're looking for a fat bomb that's not really sweet, but isn't super savory, then this fat bomb is perfect for you. They aren't sweetened, so they rely on just the natural flavor to make them tasty.

Yields: 32

Keto, Fat Fast, Paleo Gluten-Free

Ingredients:

Truffles:

1 tsp vanilla extract

¼ tsp Himalayan salt

¼ tsp cinnamon

½ tsp green tea powder

½ c coconut milk, full fat and refrigerated

1 c coconut butter

1 c coconut oil

Coating:

1 tbsp. match green tea powder

1 c shredded unsweetened coconut

Instructions:

1. Place the above truffle ingredients into a decent size bowl. It's extremely important that your coconut oil is extremely firm, so if you need to, place it in the fridge for a bit before making these. This goes for the coconut milk as well. You don't have to use just the cream part if you want you can, but the milk needs to be firm so place it in the fridge overnight.
2. Mix everything together on high with an electric mixer. It should become fluffy and light, then place this in the refrigerator for an hour.
3. As the mixture is firming up, mix together the matcha powder and coconut and place it to the side.
4. Use a small ice cream scoop to help you turn your cold mixture into 32 balls. They should be about the size of ping pong balls.
5. Roll the truffles between your hands quickly to smooth them out then roll them into the matcha coating.
6. Place them in a container and keep these refrigerated for around two weeks.

Sea Salted Caramel

Ice cream seems to be a common weakness for people. Some feel like they have to end the day with a bowl, but it's just not a good habit to have; eating a bowl of sugar before bed. This fat bomb will provide you with something that gets your mind off the need for ice cream and provide you with healthy fats.

Yields: 10

Keto, Fat Fast, Paleo, Gluten-Free

Ingredients:

2 tsp coarse sea salt

3 tbsps. grass fed butter

1 tsp cinnamon

1/3 c cream cheese

2 tbsps. cocoa powder

½ c sunflower butter

½ c coconut oil

1 tsp vanilla

½ c heavy whipping cream

Instructions:

1. Place the whipping cream into a bowl and whip them up until it starts to form soft peaks, and then fold in the vanilla.
2. Put the cocoa powder, cream cheese, cinnamon, butter, coconut oil, and sun butter

into your food processor and mix it all up until smooth.

3. Gently fold this mixture into the cream until everything is mixed together.

4. Place the mixture into your favorite silicone mold and then top with some coarse sea salt. Place this in the freezer for six to eight hours. Pop them out and keep them in a container in the freezer.

Crave Buster

There's no magical pill you can take when trying to get healthy that will get rid of cravings, but there are steps you can take to ease the pain. If you're looking to cut out all sugars, natural and artificial, completely, then these craver buster cups will help you through the hard times.

Yields: 32

Keto, Fat Fast, Paleo, Gluten-Free

Ingredients:

1 c almond butter

1 c organic cacao powder

1 c coconut oil, melted

Instructions:

1. Once you have melted the coconut oil, whisk in the almond butter and cacao until there are no lumps.
2. Place a half of a tablespoon into 32 mini muffin cups.
3. Place the freezer or refrigerator until they are hardened.
4. Once done, keep them stored in a container in the fridge to keep them from melting.

Macaroon

Macaroons are tasty little treats full of carbs and sugar. These fat bombs take the tasty and remove the sugars to give you a keto friendly treat. These are perfect little snacks after a long day.

Yields: 10

Keto, Fat Fast, Gluten-Free

Ingredients:

3 egg whites

1 tbsp. coconut oil

1 tbsp. vanilla extract

2 tbsps. Swerve

½ c coconut, shredded

¼ c almond flour

Instructions:

1. Mix together the swerve, coconut, and almond flour.
2. Place the coconut oil in a pot and melt it. Mix in the vanilla extract.
3. Place a bowl into a freezer to help when mixing the egg whites.
4. Stir the coconut oil into the flour mixture until everything comes together.
5. Place the egg whites into the frozen bowl and whip them up into stiff peaks.

6. Gently fold the whipped egg whites into the flour, making sure not to over mix and to keep the volume of the whites.
7. Place ten even dollops of the mixture onto a baking sheet, or place them in muffin cups if you want.
8. Your oven should be at 400. Bake the macaroons for eight minutes, or until the tops begin to brown.
9. Take them out and allow them to cool. Keep the store in a container in the fridge.

Avocado and Egg

Avocado and eggs are superfoods for people on a keto diet. These are also green, so they are perfect for a St. Patrick's Day themed party. They are delicious and perfect little snacks or appetizers.

Yields: 5

Keto, Fat Fast, Paleo, Gluten-Free

Ingredients:

2 tbsps. chopped spring onions

Pepper

½ tsp salt

1 tbsp. lemon juice

¼ c mayonnaise

½ large avocado, seed removed and peeled

3 large egg yolks, cooked

Instructions:

1. Begin by hard boiling your eggs. Add a pinch of salt to your water to help keep the eggs from cracking. They should boil in water for about 15 minutes. Once done, put them in a cold water and then peel off their shells.
2. Halve your avocado and take out the seed and cut off the peel. Slice the eggs in half and then carefully take out the eggs, placing them into a bowl.
3. Slice up the avocado and put it into your food processor along with the pepper, lemon juice,

salt, mayonnaise, and egg yolks. Mix it up until it becomes smooth. If you don't have a food processor, you can also mash them with a fork until well combined.

4. You can serve this on top of cucumbers with some spring onions, or place the mixture back into the eggs whites to enjoy as a deviled egg.

Strawberry Cheesecake

These super easy fat bombs are great, especially if you love strawberries. They keep well and are perfect for a tasty snack. The best thing is, if you have heart shaped molds, then you can make cute little hearts for your sweetheart.

Yields: 12

Keto, Fat Fast, Paleo, Gluten-Free

Ingredients:

2 tbsps. heavy cream

1 tsp vanilla extract

8 drops liquid stevia – or 2 tsp Swerve – or 2 tsp coconut sugar

½ c strawberries

¼ c butter

¾ c cream cheese

Instructions:

1. Cube up the cream cheese and butter and put them in a bowl to come to room temp and soften for about 40 to 60 minutes.
2. Take a fork and mash up the strawberries and place them to the side.
3. Mix together the heavy cream, sweetener, vanilla, cream cheese, and butter using a hand mixer until they are well combined.

4. Stir the strawberries in by hand.
5. Spoon this into your candy molds and place them in the freezer for a couple of hours until they are solid.
6. Pop them out and store them in a container in the fridge.

Grasshopper Bars

Mint is my weakness, and I love having a grasshopper pie for St. Patrick's Day. Now we all have this lovely fat bomb to enjoy. It gives you the flavor of a grasshopper pie, but it doesn't have all the bad stuff in it.

Yields: varies

Keto, Fat Fast, Paleo, Gluten-Free

Ingredients:

Mint:

¾ tsp vanilla

¼ tsp salt

3/8 tsp peppermint extract

4 c shredded coconut, unsweetened

6 scoops Stevia – or coconut sugar for Paleo

¾ c coconut oil, melted

½ c sweetener – use you favorite

2 avocados

Chocolate:

1/8 tsp salt

½ tsp vanilla

½ c raw cacao powder

¼ c sweetener – use your favorite

½ c coconut oil

Instructions:

1. Grease up an eight by eight baking dish.
2. Place all of the above ingredients for the mint layer into your blender and mix it up until it is smooth. If you want to have the coconut texture, then don't process until it is completely smooth.
3. Place this across the bottom of your prepared dish and slide it into the freezer until hardened.
4. Meanwhile, place the sweetener and coconut oil in a pot and heat until it is melted and combines.
5. Take it off the heat and mix in all the other chocolate layer ingredients, mixing until well combined.
6. Pour this mixture over your frozen mint layer. Return this to the freezer so that your chocolate layer can become hard.
7. Slice into squares and then place them into a container that should be kept in the freezer or the refrigerator.

Chocolate

Chocolate is one of the best parts of Easter. Kids load up on it, and the parents snitch it while they sleep at night. These fat bombs will prevent you parents from stealing your children's candy and feeling guilty for it.

Yields: 14

Keto, Fat Fast, Gluten-Free

Ingredients:

35 g walnut halves

2 tbsps. tahini paste

1 tbsp. sweetener of choices

25 g cocoa powder, unsweetened

125 g coconut oil

Instructions:

1. Heat the coconut oil up until it is melted.
2. Place the rest of the ingredients, except for the walnut halves, into the coconut oil. Mix it all together and stir it often until it cools off a bit. This will keep the ingredients from sinking to the bottom.
3. Pour this mixture into an ice cube tray and place it in the fridge until they are semi hard.
4. Squish a walnut into the top of each of the bombs and set it back into the fridge to set completely.
5. Pop them out of the tray and then store them in the fridge.

Almond Pistachio

The longer you are on a paleo or keto diet, the less likely you are to crave sweets. This is a good thing though. So for those of you who have already reached that point, I give you these fat bombs

Yields: 36

Keto, Fat Fast, Paleo, Gluten-Free

Ingredients:

¼ c raw pistachios, chopped

¼ tsp Himalayan salt

¼ tsp almond extract

2 tsp chai spice

1 tbsp. vanilla extract

¼ c ghee

½ c coconut milk, full fat and chilled

1 c coconut oil, firm

1 c coconut butter

1 c almond butter

½ c cacao butter, chopped and melted

Instructions:

1. Grease up a square baking dish and then place on the parchment paper, let it overhang the edges to help you remove it easily.

2. Place the cacao butter in a pot and melt, or you can melt it in the microwave. Make sure you often stir no matter how you melt it.
3. Put all of the above, minus the pistachios and cacao butter, into a bowl. Use a hand mixer to mix everything up, slowly moving from low to high speed. Do this until everything becomes airy.
4. Place the cacao butter into the almond mixture and start mixing again until it is incorporated well.
5. Place this into your prepared pan and spread it out. Add the pistachios over the top.
6. Place in the fridge for around four hours, or overnight.
7. Slice these into 36 squares and keep stored in a container and in the fridge.

Summer

Savory Salmon

Most fat bombs tend to be a sweet treat, but not this one. This little bit is savory and helps those that don't like consuming artificial sweeteners. These treats can be eaten on lettuce or low carb bread.

Yields: 6

Keto, Paleo, Fat Fast, Gluten-Free

Ingredients:

Pinch salt – optional

1 to 2 tbsps. dill, chopped

1 tbsp. lemon juice

½ package smoked salmon

1/3 c butter, grass-fed

½ c cream cheese, full fat

Instructions:

1. Put the salmon, cream cheese, and butter into your food processor.
2. Sprinkle with the chopped dill and the lemon juice. Pulse the mixture until it comes together and turns smooth.
3. Place some parchment paper on a baking sheet and then dollop little rounds of the mixture. They should be about two and a half tablespoons per bomb. Sprinkle some extra

dill on top and slide into the fridge for a couple of hours.

4. You can also just spoon everything into a container and eat now or keep refrigerated for a week. When serving spoon two and a half tablespoons of the mixture out per serving. Enjoy with lettuce or low carb bread.

Bacon and Guacamole

Fat bombs may not be necessary for everyone on a keto or low carb diet, but they are sure great to have on hand if needed. If you're somebody on a fat fast, then they are pretty much your energy source. These fat bombs will take you south of the border. It eliminates the tomatoes from the guacamole just so that they don't become watery, but it does add bacon.

Yields: 6

Keto, Paleo, Fat Fast, Gluten-Free

Ingredients:

4 slices bacon

1 to 2 tbsps. cilantro, chopped

¼ tsp salt

Cayenne or black pepper

1 tbsp. lime juice

½ small onion, diced

1 chili pepper, chopped

2 garlic cloves, crushed

¼ c ghee softened

½ large avocado

Instructions:

1. Your oven should be set to 375. Place parchment paper onto a baking sheet and lay the bacon strips across it, making sure not to overlap them. Put the bacon in the oven and bake around ten to 15 minutes, or until it is browned. The time it takes to cook will depend on how thick your bacon is. Once done, place to the side so they can cool down.

2. Take the half of avocado and add in the pepper, salt, lime juice, cilantro, garlic, chili pepper, and butter and mash them all together. Adjust the pepper and salt to your taste.

3. Once mashed, mix in the onion and combine well.

4. Take the bacon grease of the baking sheet and pour it into the guacamole and stir it in. Place foil over the bowl and place in the fridge for 20 to 30 minutes.

5. Crumble up the bacon into tiny pieces for the "breading." Take the guacamole out and form into six balls. A spoon or an ice cream scoop can help to make the balls. Roll your balls into the back, pressing it into the ball to stick. Place on a tray that you can slide into the fridge.

6. Once hard, store in a container and keep refrigerated.

Sunbutter

Sunbutter, a healthy fat that also makes you think about the beach when you hear it. This mix with lots of other tasty and healthy ingredients will put those summer cravings at bay.

Yields: varies

Keto, Fat Fast, Gluten-Free

Ingredients:

½ c raisins

2 c shredded coconut, unsweetened

¼ c raw cacao powder

2 drops liquid stevia

1 tbsp. vanilla extract

1 c sunflower butter

2 tbsps. cocoa butter

1/3 c coconut oil

Instructions:

1. Place the sunflower butter, coconut oil, and cocoa butter into a pot and let it all melt together.
2. Place in the cacao powder, vanilla, and stevia and mix well.
3. Fold in the raisins and the coconut until well distributed.
4. Pour this batter into silicon molds. The amount you get will depend on the size of

molds you have. You can also pour it into a square baking dish with parchment paper.

5. Place in the freezer and let it set up.
6. Remove the fat bombs from the mold or cut them into squares if you used a baking dish.
7. Place in the storage container and keep them in the fridge or freezer.

Blueberry Bliss

During the summer you can get all the fresh produce you want cheaper than you can anytime of the year. Plus it's fresher and contains more nutrients. Overall, it just seems to taste better to bite into a blueberry in the summer than the winter.

Yields: 24

Keto, Paleo, Fat Fast, Gluten-Free

Ingredients:

¼ to ½ tsp stevia – or coconut sugar if Paleo

½ c coconut butter

1 c coconut oil

14 oz blueberries, frozen

2 c raw cashews, soaked for two hours

Instructions:

1. Place the blueberries into a bowl and microwave them for around a minute so that they warm up.
2. Place all of the above ingredients, including the blueberries, into your food processor and mix them up until they are well incorporated.
3. Place in a bowl and let them freeze for about 30 minutes.
4. Take the bowl out and use your hands to make the mixture into little balls.
5. Put them in a pan and place them in the freezer for another 30 minutes to help them set up. A cookie sheet works the best so that the balls don't stick together.
6. Keep them stored in a container and in the fridge.

Neapolitan

The three most popular ice cream flavors are vanilla, strawberry, and chocolate. There are lots of people out there that love to have all three in one. This fat bomb is here to give you just that but packed full of healthy fats. This may be a little time consuming, but in the end, it's worth it.

Yields: 24

Keto, Fat Fast, Gluten-Free

Ingredients:

2 strawberries

1 tsp vanilla extract

2 tbsps. cocoa powder

25 drops liquid stevia

2 tbsps. erythritol

½ c cream cheese

½ c sour cream

½ c coconut oil

½ c butter

Instructions:

1. Place the liquid stevia, erythritol, cream cheese, sour cream, coconut oil, and butter into a bowl. With an immersion blender, mix everything together until it becomes smooth.
2. Split this mixture into three different bowls. To one bowl add in the cocoa powder, to

another bowl add the strawberries, and to the last bowl add the vanilla.

3. Use your immersion blender again to mix the three different mixtures thoroughly. The immersion blender will help to break up the strawberries. Pour the chocolate mixture into a glass measuring cup.

4. Pour the chocolate mixture into the bottom of 24 square silicone molds. Place this in your freezer for 30 minutes to set up.

5. Place the vanilla into the glass measuring cup and pour onto of the chocolate. Slid it into the freezer for another 30 minutes.

6. Finish it up by doing the same thing with the strawberry mixture. Freeze this time for an hour.

7. Once they're set, take them out of the molds and enjoy. Keep stored in the fridge.

Strawberry Cheesecake

These lovely little bites taste just like a strawberry cheesecake, something that is typically off limits for a person following a low carb diet. You can easily adjust this if you are dairy intolerant and use coconut milk instead of cream cheese, and then the coconut oil instead of the butter.

Yields: 12

Keto, Fat Fast, Gluten-Free

Ingredients:

½ c strawberries, fresh

¾ c cream cheese softened

¼ c butter softened

2 tbsps. powdered erythritol

1 tbsp. vanilla extract

Instructions:

1. Put the butter and cream cheese into a bowl. Set it on the counter for 30 to 60 minutes so that the mixture softens up. The butter needs to be softened; otherwise, it will be hard to mix.
2. Clean up the strawberries and remove the greens. Put them in a bowl and mash them up with a fork. You can also place them in a blender if you want them smoother.
3. Mix the vanilla and erythritol in with the strawberries. Check to make sure all the other

ingredients have reached room temp before adding in the strawberries.

4. Place the strawberries in with the cream and butter. Use a hand mixer, and combined the ingredients until smooth.

5. Spoon this into silicon muffin molds, or some candy molds, whichever you want. Place them in the freezer for around two hours, or until they have firmed up.

6. Once they are done, pop them out and keep them in a container in the freezer.

Cheesy Jalapeno

People with a busy life often live off of fat bombs and snacks to help them through the day. If you're trying to reduce the amount of sweets you eat, even low carb, then these savory bites will be able to help you out. These fat bombs will remind you of the famous jalapeno poppers appetizer.

Yields: 6

Keto, Fat Fast, Paleo, Gluten-Free

Ingredients:

2 g jalapeno peppers, deseeded and chopped

¼ c cheddar or gruyere, shredded

4 slices bacon

¼ c ghee or butter, unsalted

3.5 oz cream cheese, full fat and softened

Instructions:

1. Place the ghee and cream cheese in a bowl and mash them together. You can also place them in a food processor and mix.
2. Your oven should be at 325.
3. Place parchment paper on a rimmed baking sheet, this will help to catch the bacon grease that you will use later on.
4. Place the bacon on the baking sheet, making sure that it doesn't overlap.
5. Bake them in the oven for 25 to 30 minutes or until they have crisped up. The cooking time will vary on how thick your bacon is.

6. Take them out and let them cool. Once you can handle them, crumble it up into a bowl and place it to the side until you use it.
7. Mix the bacon grease, jalapenos, and cheese into the creamed mixture. Make sure it is well combined. Place in the refrigerated for around an hour to allow it to set up.
8. Separate the mixture into six balls and set them on a plate with parchment paper. Roll them into the bacon, pressing it down to make sure the bacon sticks. Keep in a container in the fridge.

Lemon

These tart little treats are like a burst of sunshine in your mouth. They are sweet yet sour, and the perfect snack to boost your energy and attitude during the middle of the day. They are also full of MCTs to fight off diseases.

Yields: 16

Keto, Fat Fast, Gluten-Free

Ingredients:

Pinch salt

2 to 4 tbsps. erythritol, powdered

1 to 2 lemons, zest

¼ c coconut oil softened

7.1 oz coconut butter, softened

Instructions:

1. First, you need to zest your lemons and ensure that the coconut oil and coconut butter has softened to room temperature. Using a fine grater for the zest will make sure that you don't get large pieces of peel.
2. Place all of the above ingredients into a bowl and mix everything together. You want to make sure that the sweetener and the zest are evenly distributed throughout.
3. Grab a candy mold, silicone mold, or mini muffin cups and fill them with a tablespoon of the mixture. Set onto a tray that you can slide into your fridge.

4. Refrigerate them for 30 to 60 minutes, or until they have become solid.
5. Once they are done, remove from molds and keep stored in a container in the fridge. This will keep the coconut from melting.

Bacon Cream Cheese

These, perfect for a picnic snacks, are full of flavor and will leave you wanting more. Your friends, family, and even your kids will love these, and they won't believe they are good for you.

Yields: 8 (2 bombs per serving)

Keto, Fat Fast, Gluten-Free

Ingredients:

1 tsp garlic salt

¼ c cheddar, grated

¼ c parmesan, grated

¼ c chopped green onion

8 oz bacon, crisped and crumbled

8 oz cream cheese, softened

Crushed pork rinds

Instructions:

1. Place the parmesan, garlic, onions, bacon, and cream cheese in a bowl and mix it all together. Make sure it is well combined. Place this in the freezer for 30 minutes to harden.
2. Meanwhile, mix together the cheddar and pork rinds in a bowl.
3. Once the cream cheese has hardened up, form it into eight even balls. Roll each of them through the pork rind mixture, pressing it into the balls. Keep them stored in a container in the fridge so that the cream cheese stays hard.

Chocolate Mousse

This treat can be switched up in a blink of an eye. You can either enjoy as a mousse with a spoon or place the mixture into popsicle molds and have them as a frozen treat on a hot summer night. Either way, they are delicious.

Yields: 4

Keto, Fat Fast, Paleo, Gluten-Free

Ingredients:

Sweetener of choice to taste

1 tbsp. raw cacao powder

3 oz heavy whipping cream, whipped

2 oz cream cheese

2 oz butter, unsalted

Instructions:

1. Let the butter soften up and mix in the sweetener until it has completely come together.
2. Blend in the cream cheese until it is smooth.
3. Mix in the cacao powder until it is smooth.
4. After you whip the cream, slowly fold it into your mixture.
5. Place the mixture into cups and refrigerate, or place them in popsicle molds and set in the freezer for a frozen treat.

Ice Cream

Who doesn't love ice cream during those hot summer days? Even though the grocery store is full of flavors, brands, and levels of healthiness, you probably won't find any that has less than 15 grams of carbs, I know, I've tried. This keto ice cream fat bomb gives you a keto friendly treat that everyone will enjoy.

Yields: 5

Keto, Fat Fast, Gluten-Free

Ingredients:

8 to 10 ice cubes

8 tsp vanilla bean powder

¼ c MCT oil

1/3 c flavor variation – explained below

1/3 c xylitol

1/3 c coconut oil, melted

1/3 c cacao butter, melted

4 egg yolks

4 whole eggs

Instructions:

1. For the flavor variation you can add in a third cup of cacao powder, ground turmeric and cacao powder, mint leaves and cacao, or any other flavor variations that you can think of as long as it equals a third of a cup. You can omit it all together if you just want vanilla.

2. Place all of the above ingredients into your blender, except for the ice cubes. Blend it all together for around two minutes, until it comes together.

3. With the blender going, add in an ice cube at a time, allowing the blender to mix it in before adding another. The point is to dilute it and cool it off, so it churns better, keep adding until it is cold.

4. Place this mixture into your maker and let it churn following the directions for your machine. You can also place it into a loaf pan and put it in the freezer to freeze, stirring it every 30 minutes for the next couple of hours.

5. Keep the mixture frozen until you want to enjoy it.

Strawberry Coconut

These pureed strawberry fat bombs taste like summer in a bite. The fresh summer berries will add an extra fresh flavor to these delicious treats.

Yields: 15

Keto, Fat Fast, Gluten-Free

Ingredients:

1 tbsp. shredded coconut, unsweetened

1/3 c strawberries, diced

8 to 10 drops liquid stevia

½ tbsp. cocoa powder

1/3 c +1 tbsp. coconut oil

1/3 c coconut butter

Instructions:

1. Put the stevia, cocoa powder, 1/3 cup coconut oil, and the coconut butter into the top of a double boiler. Stir often and cook until it is completely melted and mixed together.
2. In another skillet, place the strawberries and couple of spoonfuls of water in and mix. Let it cook until the strawberries soften. Mash the strawberries up with a fork. Place the strawberries and a tablespoon of the melted coconut oil into your blender along with some stevia. Blend it up until smooth.
3. Place the coconut mixture into some candy molds. Place a teaspoon of the strawberries

into each of the fat bombs. Add a little bit of coconut over top of them.

4. Put these in the fridge to harden up for a few hours, then remove them and keep in a container in the fridge.

Daily Greens

What could be better than having a fat bomb full of healthy fats, but a fat bomb full of greens and fat? A little boost of healthy nutrients is good for everybody, especially people that eat a diet that eliminates some of the natural sources of nutrients. This fat bomb use keto friendly green powders.

Yields: 14

Keto, Fat Fast, Paleo, Gluten-Free

Ingredients:

½ c coconut oil, room temp

2 tbsps. greens+ O powder, vanilla – or favorite green powder

1 ½ c shredded coconut, unsweetened

For chocolate:

¼ c cacao powder

Instructions:

1. Place parchment onto a baking sheet and place it to the side. If you want to add a topping, place extra coconut or hemp hearts into separate bowls.
2. Place the greens powder and the coconut into your stand mixer bowl, or your food processor. Mix it up until the greens have covered the coconut. Mix in the coconut oil
3. Continue to mix until everything starts to hold together.

4. Place a tablespoon of the dough into your hand and roll into a ball, and place it on the baking sheet. Continue until you use up the dough. This should be around 14 truffles.
5. This would be the time to roll in the toppings that you want to use. Once topped, place it in the fridge for 15 minutes.
6. Place in a container and keep it in the fridge for up to five days, or keep them frozen for 12 months.

Fall

Pumpkin Cheesecake

Everybody knows it's fall when pumpkins come out and Starbucks offers pumpkin spice latte, so let's bring that iconic flavor into some fat bombs. Don't miss out on this icon flavor just because it typically comes loaded with sugar. These bites give all the flavors of fall without the guilt.

Yields: 18

Keto, Fat Fast, Gluten-Free

Ingredients:

Pinch salt

¼ c chopped pecans

½ c pumpkin puree, unsweetened

2 tsp vanilla

2 tbsps. powdered sweetener, low carb

2 tsp pumpkin pie spice

3 oz cream cheese

¼ c coconut oil

½ c butter softened

2 tbsps. coconut oil

100 g 85% dark chocolate

Instructions:

1. Use either a glass bowl set over boiling water or a double boiler, and add in the coconut oil and melted chocolate. Mix together until they come together. Take this melted mixture off the heat.
2. Grab some mini muffin cups, and drizzle 18 with this chocolate and place in the fridge for ten minutes.
3. Place vanilla, sweetener, pumpkin spice mix, cream cheese, coconut oil, and butter in a microwavable bowl and microwave for 30 seconds at a time to melt it all together.
4. Stir in the pecans and the pumpkin puree until well incorporated. Spoon this mixture into your 18 mini muffin cups. Slice this by putting it in the fridge and let it set up for around 30 minutes, or until you want to enjoy one.
5. These should stay refrigerated because the oils melt quickly. Place them in a lidded container to keep them fresh.

Prosciutto and Baked Brie

If you're somebody who doesn't like sweets, are trying to avoid sweet tasting foods, or experiences cravings after having something sweet, then a savory fat bomb will become your best friend. They eliminate the sweet flavor, yet provide you with the fat that you need. The fall inspired flavors are just a perk of these savory treats. This only serves one but is incredibly easy to increase to make more than one serving.

Yields: 1

Keto, Paleo, Fat Fast, Gluten-Free

Ingredients:

1/8 tsp pepper

6 pecan halves

1 oz Brie cheese, full fat

1 slice prosciutto

Instructions:

1. Your oven should be at 350.
2. Grab a regular muffin pan. Fold your prosciutto in half so that it looks like a square.
3. Slice this into one of the cups of your muffin tin so that it lines it all the way around.
4. Chop up the Brie into cube shapes, and keep the white skin on. Put the cheese into the cup with the prosciutto.
5. Place the pecans in with the Brie.

6. Place in the oven for 12 minutes, or until all the cheese has melted and the prosciutto has been cooked.
7. Allow this to cool for ten minutes before trying to take it out of the pan.

Pumpkin Spice

This fall flavored fat bomb is full of healthy fats and provides extra fiber with the use of flax seeds, which also helps protect people from cancer. Cinnamon also helps control blood sugar as well, so this fat bomb is an all around delicious, healthy snack.

Yields: 12 to 15

Keto, Paleo, Fat Fast, Gluten-Free

Ingredients:

¼ c Swerve, confectioner – for Paleo use ½ c coconut sugar

¼ tsp sea salt

½ tsp nutmeg

1 tsp cinnamon

1/3 c golden flax

¾ c pumpkin puree

½ c coconut oil

Instructions:

1. Place all of the above ingredients into a bowl, and mix to combine.
2. Put this mixture into your freezer for 30 minutes.
3. Take the mixture out and roll them into ball shapes and lay them out on a plate, making sure not to let them touch.
4. Place in the fridge for another hour before eating one.
5. Keep them stored in the fridge for about a week, or place them in the freezer for longer.

Caramel Apple Pie

If this flavor was in a butter or scoopable form, I could probably eat it all in one sitting. It a fat bomb form, it helps to slow down the eating process so that you don't over eat. These will take you back to the county fair with the apple pie flavor.

Yields: 23

Paleo, Gluten-Free

Ingredients:

Pinch sea salt

20 drop English toffee stevia – use raw honey if Paleo

½ c coconut butter

1 tsp cinnamon

2 tbsps. coconut oil

1 5.4 oz can coconut cream

2 organic green apples, sliced and cored

Instructions:

1. Place the coconut oils and the apples into a pan and allow them to cook until they become soft.
2. Mix in the cinnamon and make sure the apples are coated.
3. Place in all the other ingredients into your blender along with the cooked apples and puree them up until smooth.
4. Place the mixture into some silicon molds of your choosing.

5. Place them into the freezer until they become hard. Remove them from the molds and place them into a plastic bag and keep them refrigerated.
6. Make sure you don't eat them in one sitting.

Cinnamon Butter

Consuming grass-fed butter should be part of your daily diet because it's full of nutritional benefits. So unless you're intolerant to dairy, you should add more grass-fed butter. Luckily, this fat bomb will help you add that butter into your diet as well as some tasty cinnamon.

Yields: varies

Keto, Fat Fast, Paleo, Gluten-Free

Ingredients:

Salt – if using unsalted butter

1 ½ tsp vanilla

1 tbsp. cinnamon

¼ c raw honey

1 lb grass-fed butter

Instructions:

1. Set your butter out on the counter to let it soften. You should be able to squish it some with your finger.
2. Place the vanilla, honey, cinnamon, and butter in your food processor. Mix it up for a few minutes to mix everything together and to whip up the butter a little bit. Stop when you need to for scraping the sides down to make sure everything is mixed together well.
3. Spoon this mixture into your silicone molds. If you don't have a mold, you can place

parchment on a baking sheet and place dollops of the mixture onto it.

4. Place this in the freezer for a couple of hours for it to set up. Take them out of the mold or off the parchment and place into a storage container and keep them in your freezer.

Cream Cheese Clouds

Another name for these is ghost poo, once you make them you will see what I mean. That means these are perfect to make around Halloween as a treat for your friends. These little white swirls of goodness will help to feel that hungry hole you may experience.

Yields: 24

Keto, Fat Fast, Gluten-Free

Ingredients:

½ tsp vanilla

¾ c Splenda

½ c butter, unsalted and softened

8 oz cream cheese, softened

Instructions:

1. Place in a bowl and beat it up until it becomes fluffy.
2. Place bit sized pieces onto a baking sheet lined with wax paper. You can also place it in a sandwich bag, snip the tip off and pipe it out.
3. Place in the freezer for an hour, or until it has firmed up.
4. Keep this stored in the freezer.

Coconut Oil

Coconut oil contains MCTs, which are medium chain triglycerides. The body is able to utilize these easy to help fight against things such as heart disease. It's also extremely versatile to use and can be used in place of most oils. So these fat bombs are healthy, delicious, and quick to through together.

Yields: 14

Keto, Fat Fast, Paleo, Gluten-Free

Ingredients:

½ tsp vanilla bean powder – optional

4 oz raw chocolate chips

2 tbsps. raw honey

1/3 c coconut oil, melted

2 c unsweetened coconut, shredded

Instructions:

1. Place the vanilla bean powder, raw honey, coconut oil, and shredded coconut into your blender. Mix it up until everything comes together and becomes crumbly.
2. Place wax paper onto a plate or a baking sheet. Take a tablespoon and scoop out the mixture, forming into a ball with your hands. Place it on the wax paper. Continue until you use all the mixture. Put the balls in the freezer for ten minutes.
3. Use your favorite method of melting chocolate, and melt the chocolate chips until they are

smooth. Take a butter knife and drizzle the chocolate over the coconut balls. Put them back in the fridge to set the chocolate for ten minutes. Keep them stored in a container in the fridge.

Almond Joy

If you find yourself missing your favorite candy bars, then fat bombs are where you should look. You can typically find any candy bar in fat bomb form. These almond joy fat bombs taste like the real thing but are full of healthy fats, so there is zero guilt.

Yields: 12

Keto, Fat Fast, Gluten-Free

Ingredients:

Filling:

¼ tsp xanthan gum

½ tsp almond extract

20 drops liquid stevia

2 tbsps. coconut oil

¼ c canned coconut milk

1 c coconut flakes

Coating:

12 almonds

20 drops liquid stevia

4 tbsps. coconut oil

2 oz bakers chocolate, unsweetened

Instructions:

1. For the filling, place the coconut milk in a pot and heat up.
2. Mix in the coconut flakes and the coconut oil and mix it all together, letting it cook down a little bit.
3. Stir in the almond extract and the stevia drops. Let it all cook together for about five minutes.
4. Mix in the xanthan gum
5. Place parchment paper into an eight by four loaf pan and pour the mixture in. Press it out to a half inch thickness and place it in the fridge for an hour.
6. Pull the paper out and slice it into 12 pieces, as evenly as you can get them.
7. Press an almond onto the top of each of the squares and slide them back in the freezer until the coating is made.
8. For the coating, chop up the chocolate and place it in a bowl that can be put in the microwave.
9. Place in the stevia and the coconut oil. Microwave everything until it is melted completely. Stirring often to incorporate it together.
10. Take the bars out of the freezer and dip the tops in the coating or drizzle the coating over them.
11. Keep them stored in the fridge for a snack.

Pecan Pie

It wouldn't be fair to watch everybody else enjoying a slice of pecan pie that you can't have. These fat bombs will give you something just as good, and leave your family jealous of the bit sized portions.

Yields: 10

Keto, Fat Fast, Paleo, Gluten-Free

Ingredients:

1 tsp vanilla

2 tbsps. Zen sweet – sweetener of choice

¼ c heavy cream

3 tbsps. butter

2 oz. sugar-free chocolate, chopped

1 c chopped pecans

Instructions:

1. Place the butter into a pot and brown it up. Make sure you often stir so that it doesn't end up burning.
2. After it becomes golden quickly mix in the heavy cream. Lower the heat so that it just simmers.
3. While stirring quickly, add the vanilla and your sweetener of choice. Make sure you break up any lumps that want to form.
4. Stir constantly for the next five minutes as everything starts to thicken.

5. Once it reaches a consistency of caramel and is a little bit darker, take it off the heat.
6. Stir in the pecans immediately, and then place spoonfuls of the mixture onto trays that have been lined with parchment. It should make around ten clusters depending on their sizes.
7. Set them in the freezer for five minutes.
8. Place the dark chocolate in the microwave for a few seconds to melt it. Drizzle the chocolate over the clusters.
9. Place in a container and keep them stored in the fridge.

Maple Almond Fudge

These tasty little bites will take you from convincing yourself to cheat so that you can have something sweet, to have a treat that won't hurt your diet. This has all the perfect fall flavors wrapped into one, and you'll think you're doing a bad thing by eating them.

Yields: 24

Keto, Fat Fast, Paleo, Gluten-Free

Ingredients:

1 tbsp. maple syrup, zero carb or organic

2 tbsps. coconut oil

¼ c butter

½ c almond butter

Instructions:

1. Place the coconut oil, butter, and almond butter in a bowl and microwave for 30-second intervals until they are melted and completely mixed together.
2. Stir in the maple syrup and mix well.
3. Mini muffin liners into a mini muffin tin and pour the mixture inside of the liners.
4. Place in the freezer or fridge until they are hard.
5. Keep these in a container in the fridge for a firm consistency.

Pumpkin Pie Bites

Pumpkin is everywhere in the fall, and no Thanksgiving or Halloween is complete without some. These tasty little bites will give all the taste of your favorite pie with the added sugars.

Yields: 15

Keto, Fat Fast, Paleo, Gluten-Free

Ingredients:

½ c pecans

2 tsp pumpkin pie spice

¼ c erythritol – or favorite sweetener

½ c coconut oil

2 oz coconut butter

½ c pumpkin puree

Instructions:

1. Begin by melting your coconut oil if it's not already in a liquid state. Get the coconut butter melted down as well so that it is soft and can be worked with easier.
2. Mix together the coconut oil, coconut butter, and pumpkin puree until it is well combined.
3. Mix in your choice of sweetener. Then stir in the pumpkin pie spice.
4. After everything has been well combined, place it into your containers. An ice cube tray or candy molds work well.

5. Place the pecans in a dry skillet and toast them up until fragrant. You don't have to do this, but it helps to bring out the nuttiness of the pecan.
6. Place the pecans on the fat bombs, pressing them slightly down so that they stick.
7. Place them in the refrigerator until solid. Remove them and store in a container in the fridge.

Blackberry Coconut

These fat bombs won't kick you out of ketosis if that's your goal, and will also help curb any cravings you may be having. They also come out a pretty color that would make any table scape look pretty for the fall holidays.

Yields: 16

Keto, Fat Fast, Paleo, Gluten-Free

Ingredients:

1 tbsp. lemon juice

¼ tsp vanilla powder

½ tsp stevia drops

½ c blackberries, frozen or fresh

1 c coconut oil

1 c coconut butter

Instructions:

1. Put the blackberries, if frozen, coconut oil, and coconut butter into a saucepan and heat up with mixing everything together.
2. Place the melted coconut mixture, along with all the other above ingredients, into your blender and mix it up until smooth. Let the coconut oil mixture cool slightly because if it's warm, it can cause some separation.
3. Place parchment in a square pan and pour the mixture into your pan.
4. Place it in the fridge until it is hard.
5. Take out the fat bomb and slice them into 16 squares.
6. Keep these stored in the fridge in a container.

Coconut Candies

These basic fat bombs are delicious and healthy. If you're not looking for fancy flavors, special ingredients, or anything off the wall, these are for you.

Yields: varies

Keto, Fat Fast, Gluten-Free

Ingredients:

Desiccated coconut – for rolling

2 tbsps. almond butter

2 to 4 tbsps. cocoa powder, unsweetened

½ tsp sea salt

1 to 2 tbsps. sweetener, your choice

1 tsp vanilla

1 c coconut oil, softened

Instructions:

1. Place all of the above into the bowl of your food processor and mix it up until completely smooth.
2. Place tablespoon drops onto a baking sheet that has parchment paper on it. Roll them in coconut if you want to at this point.
3. Place the candies in the fridge until they are solid, and then keep them refrigerated.

Winter

White Chocolate Butter Pecan

There's no typo there, white chocolate in a low carb fat bomb. Cocoa butter is an amazing tool for fat bombs, and with a little added sweetener, like erythritol turns it into white chocolate. Then the next thing is to figure out what flavor to mix with it, so what better flavor to mix into white chocolate than butter pecan. Never knew this famous ice cream flavor would be great for a low carb treat. These tasty bombs are great for an end of the day treat.

Yields: 8

Keto, Gluten-Free, Fat Fast

Ingredients:

½ c chopped pecans

Pinch salt

Pinch Stevia

¼ tsp vanilla extract

2 tbsps. erythritol, powdered

2 oz cocoa butter

2 tbsps. butter

2 tbsps. coconut oil

Instructions:

1. Place the butter, coconut oil, and cocoa butter in a pot and melt it all together. Turn the heat off once mixed.
2. If you don't actually have powdered erythritol, it's fairly simple to make. Put your regular erythritol into a small blender or NutriBullet and pulse it up until it forms a powder. Mix two tablespoons of this into the melted butter mixture until it comes together.
3. Mix in a pinch of salt to help the sweetness come out.
4. Now mix in the optional Stevia. There are people that say it helps to work against the cooling effects of erythritol.
5. Stir in the vanilla extract.
6. Get your candy molds or silicone cupcake molds. Add some of the pecans to each of the molds, and three or four pecans in each should work, but you do what you want. Also, hazelnuts and walnuts are great alternatives if you don't have any pecans.
7. Place the white chocolate mixture into each of the molds, covering the nuts. Slide this immediately into the freezer.
8. Let this freeze around 30 minutes. They need to be really cold before eating because they will melt easily. Keep them refrigerated or frozen.

Chocolate Cherry

If you are someone like me, then you love those cordial cherries that come out around the holidays. Unfortunately, they aren't all that healthy, and it's hard to keep from eating the whole container in one sitting. So this recipe is here to provide with something just as good but is also good for you.

Yields: 12

Keto, Fat Fast, Gluten-Free

Ingredients:

¾ c frozen sweet cherries, thawed

½ tsp vanilla extract

½ tsp almond extract

5 drops stevia

3 tbsps. cacao powder

¼ c coconut butter, melted

¼ c coconut oil, melted

Instructions:

1. If you have never melted coconut butter, the best way to do so is to boil a pot of water and stick the glass jar into it. Stir it often and keep an eye on it. This will prevent uneven cooking when trying to melt it in the microwave.
2. Place all of the above ingredients into a bowl, except for the cherries, and mix together.
3. Mash up the thawed cherries using a fork. Stir the cherries and the juices into the chocolate.

4. Place a tablespoon of the mixture into mini cupcake liners, or you can use an ice cube tray. Place them in the freezer to set up.
5. Once set, place in a storage container and keep them stored in the refrigerator.

Red Velvet

Christmas, red velvet cake, cream cheese icing, I can feel my waistline expanding. No worries though, these fat bombs will give you the deliciousness of the cake with the unhealthy parts. It's best if you use a beetroot based food coloring to keep it natural.

Yields: 24

Keto, Fat Fast, Gluten-Free

Ingredients:

1/3 c heavy cream, whipped

4 drops red food coloring, natural

1 tsp vanilla

3 tbsps. natvia

3.5 oz butter

4.4 oz cream cheese

35. 90% dark chocolate, sugar-free

Instructions:

1. Place the chocolate into a glass or metal bowl and set it over a pot filled with simmering water. If the bowl touches the water, it may burn the chocolate. Stir often.
2. As the chocolate is melting, stir together all the rest of the above ingredients using a hand mixer. You should mix for three minutes on medium so that everything is mixed well.

3. Turn the speed to low, and slowly pour in the melted chocolate. Mix for another two minutes.

4. Place the batter into a piping bag and pipe circles of the mixture onto a baking sheet lined with parchment paper. Place this in the fridge for at least 40 minutes to set up. Top with whipped cream.

Peppermint

Winter and peppermint are the perfect combos. These treats are a great way to curb a sweet craving, and they give you a burst of freshness. These get rid of feeling like you have to have a high carb snack.

Yields: 6

Keto, Fat Fast, Paleo, Gluten-Free

Ingredients:

2 tbsps. cocoa, unsweetened

¼ tsp peppermint extract

1 tbsp. sweetener – your choice

125 g coconut oil, melted

Instructions:

1. Combine the peppermint, sweetener, and melted coconut oil together.
2. Place this mixture into half of a silicon mold, don't fill them up to the top, and make sure you only use half of the mixture, there is going to be another layer. Place this in the fridge to set up.
3. Mix the cocoa into the rest of the coconut oil mixture. Once it's well combined, pour this on top of the white layer.
4. Place this back into the fridge to set up completely. Pull them out and store them in a container. They should be kept in the fridge.

Peanut Butter Fluff

It's hard to think of something tasting delicious and it being low in carbs and full of healthy fats. This fat bomb is here to prove that it is possible. It literally only takes a few minutes to make, but it does tend to taste better if you give it a chance to refrigerate overnight.

Yields: 8

Keto, Fat Fast, Gluten-Free

Ingredients:

½ square unsweetened chocolate

3 to 4 packets stevia

½ tsp vanilla extract

2 tbsps. peanut butter

4 oz cream cheese

½ c heavy whipping cream

Instructions:

1. Place the whipping cream into a bowl and whip it up until it starts to form stiff peaks, then place it to the side.
2. Cream the stevia, vanilla, peanut butter, and cream cheese together in a different bowl.
3. Place the cream cheese into the bowl with the whipped cream, and mix them together until they are fluffy.
4. Grate the square of chocolate over the top.
5. For best results, keep the mixture refrigerated.

Fudge

I don't know about you, but the holiday isn't complete without some of my Grandmother's fudge, but unfortunately, it is full of carbs and sugar. Luckily, this fat bomb is to the rescue. Instead of carbs, it's full of healthy fats to keep you full and curb cravings.

Yields: 12 – depending on size

Keto, Fat Fast, Paleo, Gluten-Free

Ingredients:

Pinch salt

¼ tsp powdered stevia – or 1 tsp monk fruit sweetener

1/3 c coconut flour

½ c cocoa powder, unsweetened

1 c coconut oil

1 c nut butter

Instructions:

1. Using a pot, place in the coconut oil and nut butter and mix until they have melted.
2. Add in all the other ingredients, whisk until they completely combine
3. Place this in a bowl and put it in the freezer for 20 to 25 minutes.
4. Once the mixture has hardened up, take the bowl out and form the mixture into balls. To help you out, you should wash your hands off in cold water often and wipe them off with a

dry paper towel. This will keep from the coconut oil melting.

5. Once you have made the balls, place them on a tray and freeze for 10 to 15 minutes to harden them back up, and then you can enjoy.

6. Keep them stored in a container in the freezer.

Chocolate Chip Cookie Dough

What's not to like about vanilla, cream cheese, and chocolate chips? Nothing is better than cookie dough. It's light and fluffy, and there's something about eating these that makes you think you're doing something wrong.

Yields: 20

Keto, Fat Fast, Gluten-Free

Ingredients:

4 oz baking chips, unsweetened or stevia sweetened

1 tsp vanilla

1/3 c swerve sweetener

½ c peanut butter, or almond butter

½ c butter, salted

8 oz cream cheese, softened

Instructions:

1. Place everything into a bowl and cream them all together with a hand mixer until everything comes together. Refrigerate the dough for 30 minutes before you start scooping.
2. Grab a cookie scoop and spray it with some coconut spray.
3. Take the dough out and scoop 20 cookies out onto a baking sheet that has been lined with parchment paper.
4. Place in the freezer for another 30 minutes. Keep them stored in a container or baggies in the refrigerator.

Chocolate Coconut

The sweet, Christmas in a bite, fat bombs are full of healthy coconut oils that will satisfy that holiday sweet tooth. I've said it once, and I'll say it again, coconut oil is one of the best oils out there, and you should add as much to your diet as you can.

Yields: varies

Keto, Fat Fast, Paleo, Gluten-Free

Ingredients:

Dash of salt

2 tsp vanilla extract

6 tbsps. raw honey

½ c raw cacao powder

2 c coconut oil

Instructions:

1. Decide how hard your coconut oil is. If you keep your house cool, you may melt the oil a little bit before going ahead. If it's soft and easily scoopable, then you can probably get by with adding it straight to the food processor. If it's melted completely, place it in the fridge to get hard just a bit.
2. Place the salt, vanilla, honey, cacao powder, and coconut oil to your food processor. Mix it up until everything is well mixed, stopping to scrape down the sides if you need to.

3. Taste it at this point to see if you need to adjust any of the flavors. You can mix in more salt or honey if you need to.
4. If you have molds to place this into, then the mixture needs to be a pourable consistency. If it's a little hard, process it a little bit longer to make it thinner.
5. If you don't have molds, place parchment onto a flat surface, and the mixture should be a bit thicker so that it doesn't spread when you dollop it on the surface. If you need to, put it in the fridge for a little bit to harden it up.
6. Pour the mixture into your molds, if using, or place dollops of the mixture on your flat surface.
7. Carefully place the surface or molds into the freezer to set them up. After they are done, pop them out and place them into a container.
8. They can be kept in the freezer or fridge, but not at room temp because they will start to melt.

Snickerdoodle

Cookies are great portable desserts and perfect holiday gifts. They give you the ability to make lots of different flavors without having to decide on one specific dessert. These snickerdoodle cookies are great holiday treats and low carb snacks you don't have to feel guilty about.

Yields: 16

Keto, Fat Fast, Gluten-Free

Ingredients:

½ tsp baking soda

¾ c erythritol

Pinch salt

½ c butter, salted and softened

2 c almond flour

Coating:

1 tsp cinnamon

2 tbsps. erythritol

Instructions:

1. Your oven should be set to 350.
2. Place all of the above cookie ingredients into a bowl and mix together until it forms a stiff dough.
3. Roll this into 16 balls as close to equal in size as you can get.
4. Stir together the sweetener and the cinnamon.

5. Roll your cookie balls through the mixture to coat them well.
6. Set them on a cookie sheet and flatten them a bit with a glass.
7. Bake them for 15 minutes.
8. Allow them to cool a bit before storing them in an air tight container. They don't have to be kept refrigerated.

German Chocolate Fudge

This fat bomb will give you a delicious holiday dessert that won't cause you to fall off the keto wagon. They taste just like a German chocolate cake, but it is made of healthy fats instead of flour and sugar.

Yields: 15

Keto, Fat Fast, Gluten-Free

Ingredients:

1 c coconut, unsweetened

1 c pecans, extra for topping

Pinch salt

1 tsp vanilla

¼ c Swerve

6 tbsps. cocoa powder, unsweetened

8 oz cream cheese, softened

4 oz coconut oil, room temp

4 oz butter, softened

Instructions:

1. Your oven should be at 350. Place the pecans onto a baking sheet and bake them for six minutes.
2. Combine all the other above ingredients, minus the pecans and coconut, with a hand mixer. Whip this for around four to five minutes, or until they become fluffy.

3. Stir in the coconut and pecans. With the pecans still a little warm, it will make the batter a little loose, but this helps when you sprinkle on the extra toppings.
4. Place this into a dish that you have lined with parchment.
5. Sprinkle the top with some extra coconut and pecans.
6. Place it in the fridge to set up. Overnight typically works best, but if you want it sooner and you just can't wait, an hour will work.
7. Slice it into squares, and keep them stored in the fridge.

Peppermint Mocha

You know it's getting close to Christmas when peppermint everything starts coming out. So why not nice spice up your fat bombs with a Starbucks inspired dessert? These are full of healthy fats and happiness.

Yields: 16

Keto, Fat Fast, Gluten-Free

Ingredients:

5 to 8 drops liquid stevia

2 tbsps. cocoa powder

¼ tsp peppermint extract

3 tbsps. hemp seeds

3 tbsps. coconut oil, melted

¾ c coconut butter, melted

Instructions:

1. Combine the peppermint extract, hemp seeds, a tablespoon of coconut oil, and the melted coconut butter together.
2. Pour this mixture into molds three-quarters of the way full.
3. Place in the refrigerator until they firm up.
4. Mix together the stevia, cocoa powder, and remaining coconut oil in a bowl.
5. Drizzle this into the molds on the fat bombs.
6. Stick back in the fridge until they are completely hard.
7. Remove from the molds and keep them stored in a container in the fridge or freezer.

White Chocolate Coconut

These little treats look like little drops of snow. So whether you live in an area that gets snow or not, you can bring some snow into your life.

Yields: 24

Keto, Fat Fast, Gluten-Free

Ingredients:

Pinch salt

1 tsp coconut liquid stevia

1 tsp vanilla

½ c vanilla protein powder

1 c coconut butter

½ c coconut oil

15 oz coconut milk

4 oz cacao butter

Instructions:

1. Place the cacao butter into a pot and melt.
2. Mix in the coconut butter, coconut oil, and the coconut milk. Stir to combine; there should be no lumps.
3. Switch the heat off and stir in the salt, stevia, vanilla, and protein powder.
4. Pour this into a square baking dish that you have lined with some parchment paper.
5. Top with some extra coconut flakes if you want.

6. Place in the fridge for four hours at least to help it harden.
7. You don't have to keep these in the fridge once you cut them into squares. Keep them in an air tight container.

White Chocolate

It's not hard to hear somebody say that they didn't realize they weren't consuming enough fats to stay full. These tasty treats will make you think you're eating something that is typically full of sugar, when in fact it's made of coconut and full of good and healthy fats.

Yields: 8

Keto, Fat Fast, Paleo, Gluten-Free

Ingredients:

10 drops vanilla stevia – or favorite sweetener with vanilla extract

¼ c coconut oil

¼ c cocoa butter

Instructions:

1. Place the coconut oil and cocoa butter into a pot and let it melt while heating over low heat.
2. Set if off of the heat once they are melted and combined. Mix in the sweetener and the vanilla if using.
3. Grab eight silicone cupcake molds and pour the mixture into them. It will not fill the molds to the very top. Instead, it will probably only fill it a quarter of the way up.
4. Set them in the fridge until they harden up.
5. Take them out, and remove the fat bombs. Keep them in a container and in the fridge so that they do not melt.

Conclusion

Thanks for making it through to the end of *Fat Bombs*. Let's hope it was informative and able to provide you with all of the tools you need to achieve your goals.

The next thing for you to do is try out these recipes. There's literally enough to try a new recipe each week for the next year. Enjoy them for the energy they give you to go through the day, and impress your friends with a tasty and healthy snack.

Finally, if you found this book useful in any way, a review on Amazon is always appreciated!